Essential Oils Guide:

The Beginner's Guide Getting Started with Essential Oils for Dummies

Table of content:

Introduction - What to expect...

This book has been put together with years of experience behind it. It has been written in a way to ease you into the information you've been looking for without making you feel you need to reach for a dictionary or do further research to answer all your questions on getting started in the Aromatherapy field. This book will teach you:

• What Aromathery is and how long it's been around,
• How Aromatherapy works,
• How essential oils are made,
• How to use them safely,
• The tools, storage containers, and ingredients you will need to get you started,
• How to blend essentials oils effectively
• How to properly shop for essential oils
• How to market your product when you feel you are ready to break into selling your Aromatherapy products.

So, if you're ready to started, swipe the page and let's go…

Chapter 1 – What are Essential Oils?

In order to understand your new interest, you need to understand its origins.

Aromatherapy

Though the origins of Aromatherapy can be murky, it can be dated back to at least 6,000 years ago. They have been able to date an Ancient Egyptian papyrus to approximately 1555 BC which contained remedies for all types of sicknesses and how to apply them which are much the same applications we use today. Greeks also had a role in the history of this type of medicine. It is often said Hippocrates, the father of medicine, practiced it before it was recognized. The actual term "Aromatherapy" was coined in 1937 with a French chemist, Rene-Maurice Gattefosse, after burning himself and putting his arm in a vat of Lavender essential oil and finding that it had treated his burn. A French surgeon used essential oils during World War II to treat soldiers' wounds, further proving the potency of Aromatherapy.

Aromatherapy works by triggering the amygdala and hippocampus of the brain, the two areas that store memories emotions. When you take in the aroma, some researchers say these two parts of the brain are awakened and can influence improvements to physical, emotional, and mental health. Think of how you feel when smell cinnamon in a pie. What emotions does it trigger?

Aromatherapy is used in massage, bath, and aerosol therapies to sooth pains, anxiety and all kinds of other problems. There are a myriad of ways you can use essential oils in Aromatherapy.

How essential oils are made...

Essential oil is the most concentrated form of roots, plants, leaves, seeds, and even flower petals. Depending on the nature of the plant matter, they are made by:

-Distillation process that separates the oil from the plant.

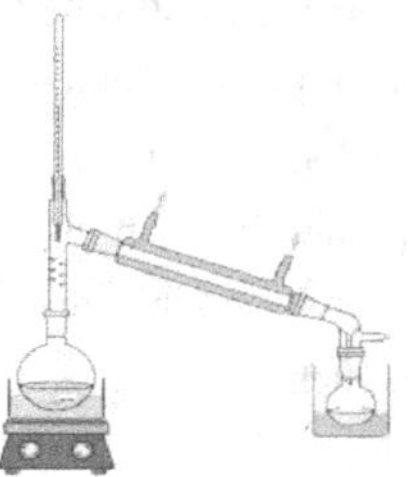

-Infusion processes

-Expressing the oil from the plant matter.

There are a few things you need to keep in mind when using essential oils.

-They can cause contact dermatitis.

When used undiluted, essential oils can cause inflammation and rashes on the contact site. For this reason, I recommend you use gloves when mixing them.

-They are highly toxic

Because of their concentrated form, it is not advised you use them undiluted unless you place them in a diffuser. They need to be kept out of the reach of children and pets.

-They are volatile.

They can evaporate easily when exposed to intense heat. Storing them in a cool, dark place can prevent this.

-They can cause side effects

There are some essential oils that can raise blood pressure, trigger allergies, and even make you more sensitive to sunlight. Make sure to properly research the essential oils before using them to avoid the side effects.

-If you have plant allergies, beware

Many plants are related to one another biologically. One example is ragweed. If you are allergic to ragweed, be leery when thinking about using any of flowers in the Chamomile family. The easiest way to avoid this is to look up the genus and species names of the plants before using them.

Chapter 2 – Tools of the Trade

Every job, hobby, or career needs proper tools, and Aromatherapy is no different. You will be surprised to find a lot of things on this list you already have in your kitchen.

Basic Tools

Glass Mixing Bowls

These are the best ones to use because the ingredients you use cannot leach any of the properties from metals or other materials used in making mixing bowls.

Food Scale

These are instrumental in accurately measuring the dry ingredients you will need to make them.

Sifter/strainer

There will be times when you will need to sift the dry ingredients to better mix them together. You can always use a strainer if you don't have a sifter or can't find one.

Measuring Spoons and cups

Like in cooking, you will need this to measure out carrier oils and other liquid ingredients you will be using.

Mixer/food processor/Mixing spoons

These are needed to properly mix dry ingredients together before adding the liquid ingredients. You can also use these to mix the liquids in with your dry ingredients.

Double boilers

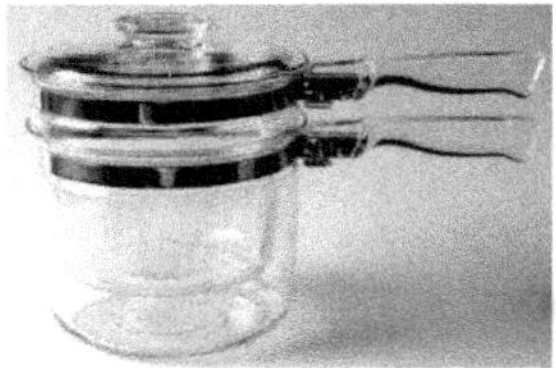

These will come in handy when melting some oils and other ingredients when they are in solid form. If you don't have one of these and can't find one, you can place a glass mixing bowl in a stock pot.

Gloves

Rubber gloves are best for mixing your essential oils.

Apron

This will help keep your clothing from being stained when mixing ingredients.

Goggles

This will keep your eyes safe from any splash back from going into your eyes.

Pipettes

This can be bought in school supply and medical supply shops. They are one-use throw-away items that can make filling tubes remarkably easy.

Dark Glass/Plastic bottles

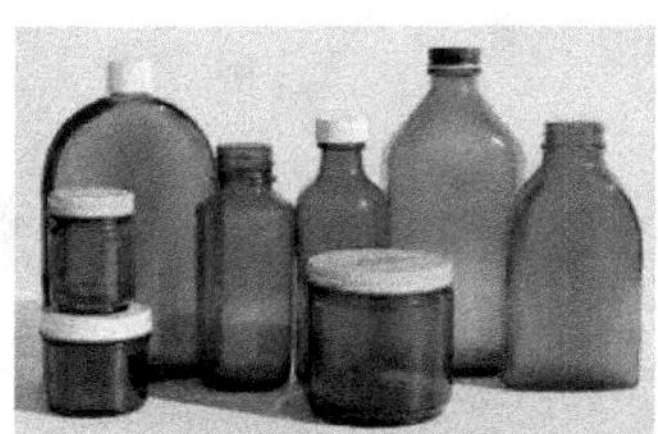

Glass is preferred because will prevent the essential oil aromas from escaping, but both will work. Dark colors, like cobalt blue and amber, will prevent sunlight from permeating into the container and reducing the product's effectiveness.

Spray Bottles

These are used for cleaners and air freshening sprays.

Labels

You will want to label your creations. The label should include the ingredients used, and expiration dates as well as uses and a name for your creation.

Recipe book/box

You will want to remember the blends you like to use the most. Keeping either a recipe box or book handy. You can also use a tablet or your computer for this, too.

Will go into the carrier oils in another chapter. This list is for the other ingredients will be needing to make all the preparations out there.

Apple Cider/White Vinegar

This is used in cleaners.

Baking Soda

This can be used in bath/mineral salts and scrubbing cleaners.

Beeswax

This is used for salves and some ointments as well as lip balms. It moisturizes and introduces vitamins as minerals to speed healing. It is also used to solidify other ingredients in preparations.

Borax

This is a naturally occurring mineral often used in mineral baths and cleaners like scrubs and laundry detergent.

Clay Powders

French and Bentonite clay powders are used in the most expensive facial masks. They help tone the skin and absorb toxins for a healthier skin tone.

Cocoa Butter

Like beeswax it is used for a therapeutic punch and a solidifying agent.

Epsom Salts

These familiar salts are used in bath salt mixtures.

Grain/clear alcohol

This is used in glass cleaners and anti-bacterial sprays. It helps in the evaporation of the other ingredients.

Lotion Base

You can purchase unscented lotion base online for making your own lotions at home.

Magnesium Flakes

This can often replace an ingredient in bath/mineral salts for extra nutritive properties.

Sea Salt

Whether white, pink, or any of the other colors on the market, these salts contain minerals beneficial for health and are used in bath and mineral salts. They are also added to cleansing scrubs for extra abrasion that doesn't scratch most surfaces.

Soap

You can by the glycerin soaps in craft stores. This is used to make personal soaps for the shower or bath and even added to recipes for laundry and other cleansers.

Washing Powders

This ingredient is added to all cleaning products. It's gentle but strong and adds extra cleaning power when needed.

Here are the many ways you can turn your essential oils into aromatherapy products. Shelf life is included with the descriptions as well as the base recipe.

Aromatherapy Sprays

These are a great way to freshen the air and lighten the mood. These last for up to a year.

-Recipe

4 Ounces of purified water
50 drops of an essential oil or EO blend

How to make it

- Blend the essential oils first
- Add the essential oils and the water to a spray bottle
- Shake well and spray.

Bath Salts/Mineral Baths

This is one of the more popular ways to use essential oils. You mix different salts with minerals and essential blends for a relaxing a therapeutic bath. These are recommended to be used when they are ready but can keep for up to six months before they start to lose their effectiveness.

-Recipe 1

1-2 Cup of Magnesium flakes or Epsom Salts
1/2 Cup of Sea Salt
10-15 Drops of an essential or EO (essential oil) blend

-Recipe 2

1 Cup Magnesium Flakes or Epsom Salts
1/4 Cup Borax
1/4 Cup Baking Soda
1/2 Cup Sea salt
10-15 Drops of an essential oil or EO blend

How to make them

• Blend the essential oils and set them aside.
• Mix the dry ingredients together after sifting them in a mixer on low. You don't need to grind the sea salt. It's better if it stays course.
• Slowly add the essential oil or blend to the dry ingredients.
• Place it in a container with a tight lid and let it sit overnight to get the most out of it.

Diffuser Blends

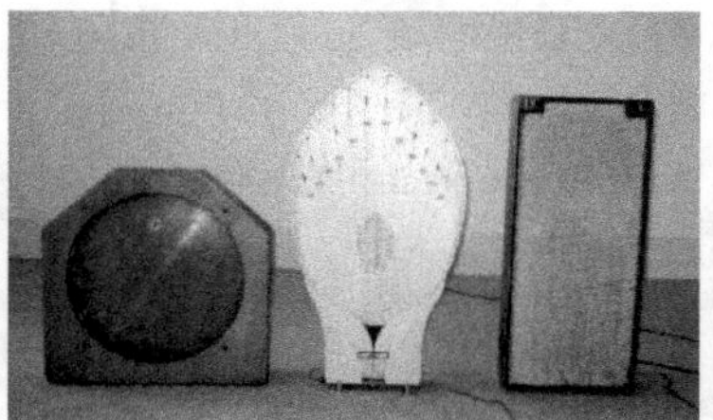

From plug-in diffusers to ones you can put in your car, they are great for dispersing the blend you make into the air. If you don't have one, you can use a candle warmer.

Essential oil blends for the diffuser can last up to two years properly stored. They are used by adding ten drops onto a candle warmer or following the directions on the diffuser you choose to purchase.

Facial Masks

Instead of paying money for a spa day (even though it's a good way to spoil yourself), you can make your own facial masks at home. When properly stored in an airtight container, the clay mixture can last for two years. The essential oil blend can last as long as the shelf life of the oil blend.

-Recipe

1 Tbsp French Clay powder
1 Tbsp Bentonite Clay powder
1 Tbsp carrier oil
12 drops of an essential oil or EO blend

Warm purified water

How to make them

• Mix the clay powder and set aside.
• Mix the essential oil blend and set aside
• Take one tablespoon of the clay and add just enough warm water to make a paste.
• Add half of the essential oil blend
• Add an even layer of the mask to the face, being careful to avoid the mouth, nostrils, and eye areas.
• Let the mask dry
• Moisten the mask with warm water.
• Scrub the face and rinse the mask off. Pat your face dry and apply moisturizer.

Glass Cleaner

Looking for a chemical free glass cleaner that really works? Here you go.

- Recipe

1/4 Cup vinegar (your choice-white or Apple Cider)
1/4 Cup Cheap clear alcohol or rubbing alcohol
1 tbsp cornstarch
2 cups water
100 drops of essential oil or essential oil blend

How to make it

• Mix all the ingredients into a spray bottle and shake until starch is dissolved.
• Shake before using as you would regular glass cleaner.

Note: If you use Tea Tree essential oil in the blend, you can use it as a sanitizing spray.

Laundry Detergent

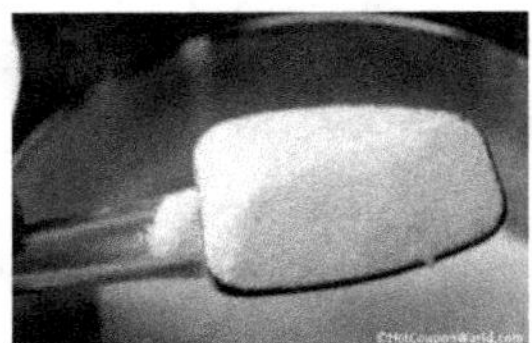

This can make large batches you can store in tightly lidded containers. It can last up to one year.

- Recipe

4 Ounces of grated bar soap, either homemade or Doctor Bronner's Castille Soap
2 parts Washing Soda
2 Parts Borax
50-75 Drops of an essential oil or EO blend

How to make it

• Mix the dry ingredients together well.
• Gradually add in the essential oil blend
• Mix in a food processor. You may need to split the essential oil blend and make more than one batch here.
• Place in a tightly lidded container.
• All you need to add is one tablespoon to a regular wash. You can Add one tablespoon of baking soda for a particularly smelly load and one tablespoon of oxyclean for an extra dirty one.

Lip Balms

This can get addictive to make once you get the hang of them. They always make more than one stick or small tin, so have plenty handy. You can pass them out to friends and family. They are good for up to six months.

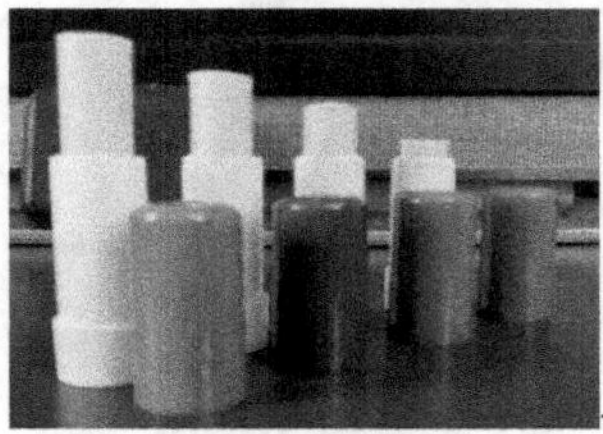

 Recipe

2 tbsp beeswax pastilles
2 tbsp shea butter
2 tbsp coconut oil
30 drops essential oil or EO blend

How to make it

• In a double boiler, place the first three ingredients.
• Stir them occasionally until they are completely melted.
• Remove the double from the heat but keep the ingredients in it to keep them from melting.
• As the mixture cools, add the essential oils.
• Use a pipette to fill the lip balm tubes.
• Wait until completely cook before capping.

Massage oils/Roll-ons

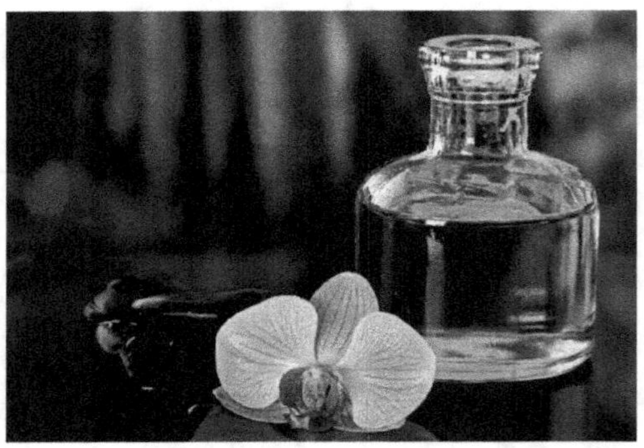

You can use massage oils to soothe tired muscles and relieve stress. The roll-on is for a more portable version of the massage oil.

- Recipe

4 Ounces of a carrier oil or carrier oil blend
50 drops of an essential oil or EO blend

How to make them.

● Mix into a dark plastic squeeze bottle or pour a small amount into a roll-on bottle.

Ointments

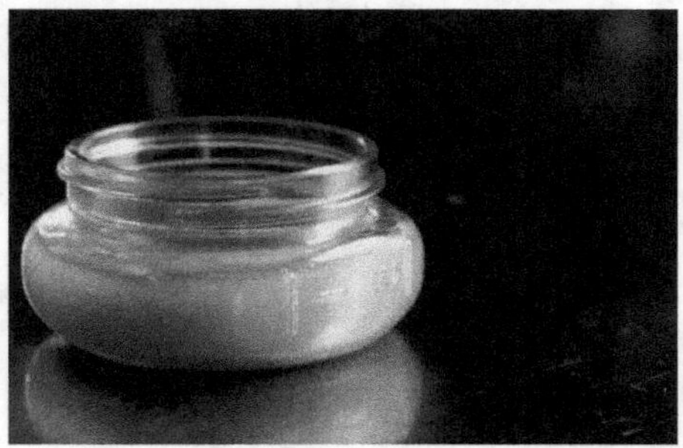

Think petroleum jelly, only there are plenty of jellies out there which act like petroleum jelly that are derived from plants.

- Recipe

2 ounces of "petroleum" jelly
25 drops of essential oil or EO blend

How to make them

- Melt the jelly in a double boiler
- Stir to make sure it melts smoothly
- Stir in the essential oil
- Place the ointment in containers and let cool before use.

Soap

You can get different types of melt-and-pour soap at hobby and craft stores or online. You will also need plastic or silicone molds to pour the soap into when you are done.

- Recipe

8 ounces of melt-and-pour soap
1 tsp essential oil or EO blend

How to make them

- Using a double boiler or crock pot, melt the soap
- Place the soap in the molds
- As the soap cools, stir in equal parts of the essential oil in each mold.
- It takes about 8 hours for the soap to harden.

Makes two 4-ouce bars.

Soft Scrub

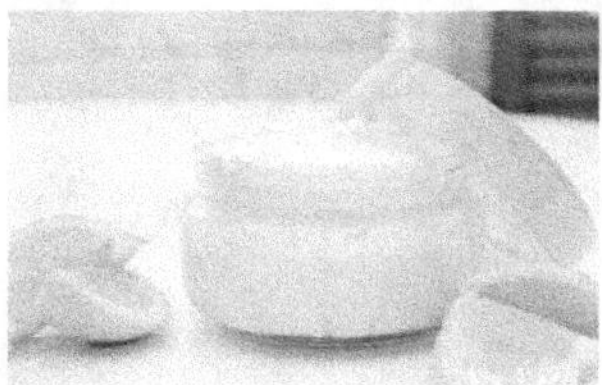

Yup, you can make that stuff you buy in the store, too.

- Recipe

1 Cup Washing Powers

1/4 Cup Borax

1/2 Cup Coarse Sea Salt

1/4 cup Apple Cider Vinegar

1/2 Cup Filtered water

2 tsp of essential oil or blend

- Mix the essentials oils first
- Add them to the vinegar. Shake well
- Add water and stir
- Mix the dry ingredients together
- In a mixer, add the liquid to the dry ingredients.

Surface Cleaner

This is something you can use for any surface and any reason. What you're using for depends on the essential oils to put in it.

- Recipe

2 cups filtered water
1/4 cup Clear alcohol or rubbing alcohol
1/4 cup Washing Powders
1/4 Cup Baking Soda
2 tsps of essential oil or EO Blend

How to make it

- Mix essential oils first
- Add essential oils to the alcohol
- Add the alcohol to the water
- Add the dry ingredients and shake until dissolved
- Use as you would any other surface cleaner

Chapter 3 – How do I blend them?

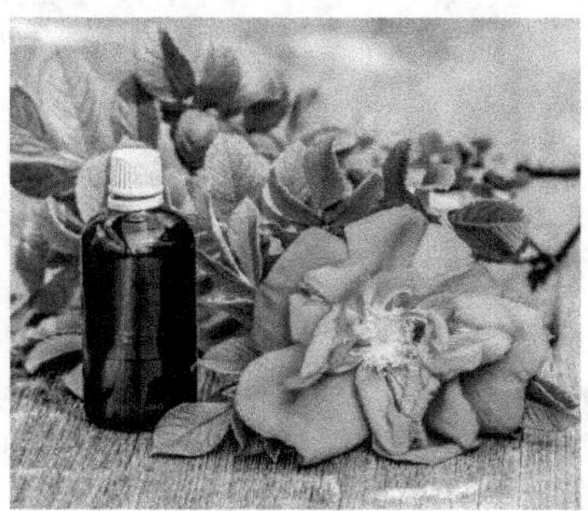

Now we get to the brass tacks of Aromatherapy, how to blend essential oils. Essential oils are classified, not only by therapeutic properties, but there evaporation rate as well. This rate is often called the "note" of the essential oil. There are three "notes".

Top note

These are the quickest to evaporate and you tend to use them in 15-25% percent concentrations in blends. By themselves, they tend to last up to about three hours. These essential oils are more commonly anti-viral, too. Here is a list of top notes:

-Bergamot (also can be middle)
-Cajuput
-Clary Sage (also middle)
-Basil (also can be middle)
-Lemongrass (also middle)

-Grapefruit
-Lemon
-Lime
-Mandarin
-Neroli (also middle)
-Niaouli
-Orange
-Eucalyptus
-Peppermint
-Petitgrain
-Hyssop
-Ravensara
-Sage
-Spearmint
-Tagetes
-Tangerine
-Tea Tree (also middle)
-Thyme (also middle)
-Verbena

Middle notes

These are the essential oils that give body and are used in concentrations of 30-40% in blends. They tend to be balancing and soothing and last up to 6 hours on their own. The middle notes are:

-Bay
-Black Pepper
-Cardamom
-Chamomile

-Cypress

-Fennel (also top)

-Juniper

-Lavender (also top)

-Marjoram

-Melissa (also top)

-Myrtle

- Nutmeg

-Palmarosa

-Pine

-Rosemary

-Spikenard

-Yarrow

Base notes

These are the essential oils that tend to be more potent and last longer. They can also be very pricey, but worth it. They are also used in concentrations of 45-55% in blends. Base notes include:

-Balsam Peru

-Cassia (also middle)

-Cedarwood

-Cinnamon (also middle)

-Clove

- Frankincense

-Myrrh

-Oakmoss

-Patchouli

-Rose

-Rosewood (also middle)

-Valerian

-Vanilla

-Vetiver

-Ylang Ylang (also middle)

For Example

If you need to make a 10 drop blend, it would look like this:

3 Drops Peppermint

3 Drops Lavender

4 Drops Sandalwood

Measuring Essential oils

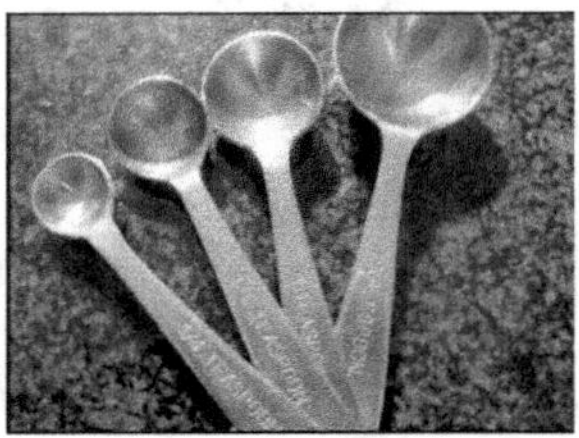

However, there will be times when you will want to make bigger batches of the blend for massage oils, soaps and the like. Here is a chart that may help with that.

1 tsp= 100 drops

3 tsp= 1 tbsp

50 drops per 4 ounces of base material/carrier oil

Carrier oils

I've mentioned these a few times already. Carrier oils are a wide variety of oils used in Aromatherapy to dilute essential oils. There are some carrier oils you can use at full strength and some you need to mix with others. There are close to 40 different carrier oils on the market. I will keep the list to the most commonly used ones.

100% Concentration

Sweet Almond

This tops the list. It is good for all skin types and is used for swelling and dry skin conditions.

It is high in essential fatty acids, vitamins E and K.

Apricot Kernel

This is another one that is widely used, often as a substitute for Sweet Almond above. It is good for all the same skin types as the oil above but also mature skin. The only nutrient that it differs in is it has no vitamin K.

Argan Oil

This is used mainly for the flaking skin, skin with sun damage, and it helps bring elasticity back to maturing skin. It is rich in the same nutrients as Almond oil.

Coconut Oil

It nourishes the skin, helps to allay itching, and is even used in hair care to help with frizz. It is rich in lauric acid. It tends to be a solid at room temperatures.

Grapeseed Oil

This oil boosts the skins natural ability to heal itself. It is recommended for combination skin or oily skin. The oil comes from the seed, and contains the same nutrients as Almond oil.

Hazelnut Oil

This oil is good for anti-aging blends, sun damage, and all types of skin as well as sensitive skin. It contains vitamin E and the Omegas 6 and 9.

Hemp Seed Oil

This oil moisturizes, soothes irritated skin, and has anti-inflammatory properties. Along with Omegas 3, 6, and 9, it has gamma linolenic acid.

Jojoba Oil

This is an odd duck for an oil as it is technically a liquid wax at room temperature. It is used for its ability to mimic sebum, one of our natural body oils. For this reason, it is recommended for mature skin types, sensitive skin, and all other skin types.

Safflower Oil

This is also a moisturizing and balancing oil. It is good for all skin types.

Sunflower Oil

This oils is also good for all skin types. It can help with dryness, irritation, combination skin, and acne.

Percentage Oils

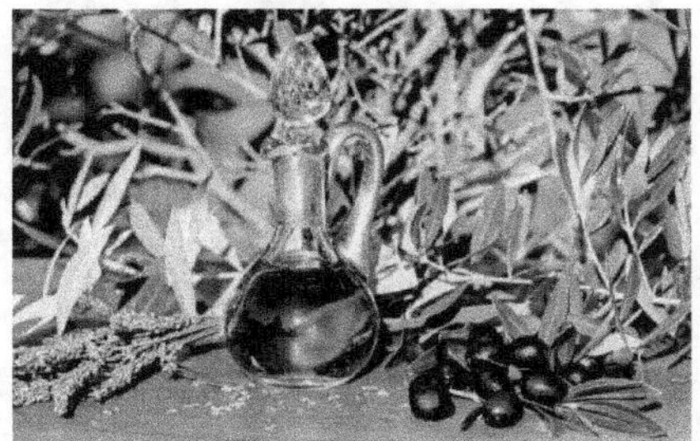

These are oils that are used in percentage concentrations either due to their pungent smell or their potency.

Avocado Oil

This softens and smooths skin. It also helps to protect it. It does suit all skin types, including mature skin. It is generally only used in 10-40% concentrations. It contains vitamins A, B, D, and E as well as Omegas 3, 6, and 9.

Evening Primrose Oil

Used in concentrations of 10-30% percent, this oil is recommended for blends that target mature skin and combination skin, but is gentle enough for all types.

Olive Oil

This is not the popular type often found in grocery stores. When shopping for this type, you are looking for the first pressing of the olives. This makes the oil a light to medium green in color. It is used in concentrations of 30-50% percent, but you will smell it the higher end. It nourishes and feeds the skin and scalp.

Sesame Oil

This oil is recommended for problem skin to help soften and smooth it. It also is helpful for sun damaged skin, mature skin, and combination skin. It is used in concentrations of 30-50%.

There are many more carrier oils out there that are lesser known. As you get more confident in your ability and knowledge of essential oils, you can look them up.

Chapter 4 – Purchasing and Selling

In every hobby or interest there are pitfalls on occasion when you purchase something and wondering how to price your skill once you are ready to sell your products.

Buyer Beware

You need to be very wary of who you choose to purchase your essential oils from and what to look for in terms of screening for purity and reputation.

Chromatography

This is a way of testing plants and oils for their purity and to see if they are contaminated. Most, if not all, reputable sellers will either list their means of purity testing or refer you to the company that they receive their plant material from and they will list the screening and testing process.

If not, contact them and ask. If they are not willing to tell you how they make sure you are getting the purest form of essential oils. Don't purchase from them.

Look out for dilutions

This is not necessarily a bad thing if you what to use a single or save money, but often times, the essential oils are pre-diluted with jojoba oil. It should say it on the label.

Be leery of low prices

We all want that bargain, but buying an essential oil that is normally pricey for way below what it should be means one of two things:

1. It's either pre-diluted or not the exact essential oil you're looking for, or
2. It's on clearance, meaning it's past its most potent, or best time to purchase it.

Either way, you are not getting what you are looking for.

Check the name, the Latin One

This is the best way to make sure you are getting the *exact* essential oil you are looking to buy. One common herb name can refer to two more plants. For example, Lavender and Spike Lavender, both are Lavender, but they are not used for the exact same thing. Check that name.

Check country of origin

There are many businesses out there that import the plants from their countries of origin to make the essential oil. The closer it is to its native land, the more potent the essential tends to be.

Getting Your Feet Wet

Now, it won't be with this book, but as you find more books with essential oil information and you start making your own blends and products, you may begin to wonder how you would set out to sell your products. Here is some advice.

Slow down

It takes hundreds of blends and product testing to make sure you have solid recipes you can use that don't smell funny or don't do exactly what you want them to. You also need to factor in how strong you want the products to be. All this takes time.

Branding

Once you have a decent list of products you want to start making, you are going to need an eye-catching logo and brand name. The name should hint at what you do so people can recognize it quickly and your logo should be memorable. After you get both of those, you can look for packaging that is right up your alley.

Business License

State laws all vary on when you should get a business license. Check your local city tax office to see what you need to get one.

Social Media

Love it or hate it, managing social media can make or break your fledgling business. There are websites and blogs out there that can help you start out on the right foot, but here are some basics:

1. You are your brand. I know this sounds elementary, but when marketing your products, all the social media accounts you open should be in your product's name. This will make it much easier for people to find you.

2. Make your pictures count! There are resources online that can help you take killer pictures of your products to make them stand out. This will help you when you open your store, too.

3. Video is king. You can make short videos displaying your process, your products, and even introducing yourself.

4. It's social media, not commercial media. Mingle; talk to people, and don't be afraid to start conversations. Just keep in mind rule 1, and you should be just fine.

Website/selling platform

There are lots of platforms you can sell your products on, Storenvy comes to mind as does Bonanza. Steer clear of Etsy. Ever since the company went public, they have allowed mass manufacturers to sell there, and that tends to drown out smaller businesses.

Policies and Guidelines

You have to sit down and write out your guidelines, shipping, and return policies. Let the customer know if they can, or how they can, make a return or exchange, if they need to do that.

Label Clearly

Remember the labels? They will be your life saver here. Don't forget to list the ingredients used on the site you use to sell your items. This will help you avoid any problems due to allergies.

Disclaimers

You need one of these, especially if you are trying to sell products that are therapeutic. Get the advice of a lawyer that is savvy in business law to help with this one. You may have to spend some money for the disclaimer, but it will be worth it in the long run.

Recommended Reading and Websites

There is a ton of information out there. To help get you started on your next step, here are some resources I often turn to:

1. The Complete Book of Essential Oils and Aromatherapy, Valerie Ann Worwood
2. The Illustrated Encyclopedia of Essential Oils, Julia Lawless
3. aromaweb.com
4. aromatherapy.com
5. The Encyclopedia of Aromatherapy, Chrissie Wildwood

Conclusion

I hope this book has given you all the basic information you will need to see if you want to delve deeper into the realm of Aromatherapy. I have also pointed you in the direction of sources I consider invaluable for either beginners or people who have been in the field a while, like myself, but don't stop there. There are forums and other sites you can check out yourself when you are more confident with your knowledge. There is a lot to learn, take in, and practice. Until next time, never stop seeking knowledge.